SUZANNE BYRD

Heart, Mind, and Hormones
The Female ADHD Experience Across Life Stages

Copyright © 2025 by Suzanne Byrd

All rights reserved. No part of this publication may be reproduced, stored or transmitted in any form or by any means, electronic, mechanical, photocopying, recording, scanning, or otherwise without written permission from the publisher. It is illegal to copy this book, post it to a website, or distribute it by any other means without permission.

First edition

This book was professionally typeset on Reedsy. Find out more at reedsy.com

Contents

1. Understanding ADHD: The Unique Female Experience — 1
2. Hormonal Influences: The Hormonal Rollercoaster — 6
3. The Impacts of ADHD on Relationships — 13
4. Career Challenges and Triumphs for Women with ADHD — 18
5. Self-Advocacy: Navigating Diagnosis and Treatment — 23
6. Mindfulness and Coping Strategies — 29
7. Body Image, ADHD & Societal Pressures — 34
8. Transitions and Life Stages: From Adolescence to Adulthood — 39
9. Community Support: Building a Network — 45
10. Embracing Your ADHD Superpowers — 51

1

Understanding ADHD: The Unique Female Experience

In a brightly lit classroom, a young girl named Sarah sat with her head down on her desk, her hair falling like a curtain around her face. The noise of pencils scratching paper and the soft hum of the teacher's voice felt distant, almost surreal. It was another day of struggling to concentrate, wrestling with a torrent of thoughts that diverted her attention from the lesson at hand. While her classmates absorbed the instructions on fractions, Sarah's mind danced from the birthday parties she wanted to plan to the vibrant colors she envisioned for them—shimmering pinks and bold yellows that made her smile. It was a kaleidoscope of creativity, bursting from her imagination like fireworks on the Fourth of July. Yet, in this vibrant mental world, the lesson about fractions left her completely behind.

As a young girl, Sarah was often praised for her creativity, her imagination, and her enthusiasm. Teachers would say, "She's such a bright student, but she just seems to lack focus," with a dismissive wave of their hands. Society celebrated her artistic abilities, yet when it came to academics, there was an undercurrent of frustration, both for herself and for her educators. Each year passed without a diagnosis, and the inconspicuous traits of ADHD slipped further under the radar, masked by societal expectations of diligence and perfection.

This is not an uncommon narrative for women with Attention Deficit Hyperactivity Disorder (ADHD). Historical and cultural biases have led many to believe that ADHD only manifests in hyperactive, disruptive behaviors typically associated with boys. Indeed, the diagnostic criteria, heavily researched and defined through predominantly male populations, have often overlooked how ADHD presents in females. Symptoms in females tend to be more internalized, making this condition particularly difficult to identify and diagnose during formative years.

The variety of ADHD symptoms range widely, from inattentiveness and distractibility to impulsivity and difficulties with emotional regulation. For girls like Sarah, invisible symptoms such as chronic procrastination, emotional overload, and an inability to work within rigid structures are common. These difficulties can be exacerbated by unrealistic societal expectations. Sarah often felt the pressure of perfection every time she entered the classroom, forcing her to place a veneer of composure over her internal chaos.

Take, for instance, the narrative of another woman, Melissa, who experienced her own journey with undiagnosed ADHD. Growing up, Melissa excelled in art but failed to see the value of her achievements in more structured academic subjects. "I just thought I was lazy or not trying hard enough," she mused in an interview years later. "Nobody really talked about ADHD for girls—it was always a boy's issue. So I internalized that lack of success as a personal failure instead." Both Melissa and Sarah represent surrogate tales for countless women who navigated their formative years with undetected ADHD.

During adolescence, when peer relationships gained immense significance, the pressure to fit into certain molds intensified. Women often find themselves deciphering complex social cues—an exhausting task for anyone, but particularly challenging for those navigating ADHD. This persistent difficulty in accessing emotional intelligence manifests itself in several ways. Women more frequently report issues with emotional regulation and social dynamics—a reality irretrievably shaped by societal constructs about femininity, cooperation, and compliance.

The repercussions of undiagnosed ADHD have lasting impacts, not only during childhood but well into adulthood. Adults like Sarah and Melissa might find themselves in endless spirals of self-doubt, reflecting on their perceived failures. Society's view of success—steady jobs, robust relationships, and academic achievements—seems unattainable amidst the ebb and flow of ADHD symptoms. Sarah, now 29, often reminisced about her childhood, realizing that her ability to hyper-focus on creative endeavors coexisted with her struggle to manage tasks as mundane as organizing her workspace or completing assignments on time.

Take a moment to consider the comparative analysis of two ADHD diagnoses: Ryan, an adolescent boy diagnosed at the age of nine, and Jennifer, a 32-year-old woman who received her diagnosis after years of silent suffering. Ryan's disruptive behavior earned him acknowledgment; he was hyperactive and impulsive in class—traits visible, not only to his teachers but also to his peers. Jennifer, on the other hand, spent years wrestling with an internal chaos no one could see. She attended therapy for anxiety, struggling silently with the frustration of being unable to complete tasks that seemed effortless for those around her.

Research supports the notion that ADHD manifests differently based on gender. In comparative studies, boys typically exhibit externalizing symptoms—acting out, displaying hyperactivity—whereas girls tend to internalize their challenges, leading to anxiety or depression. This internalization creates a cycle of self-blame; Jennifer's journey through adulthood illustrates how societal expectations could warp internal narratives and create barriers to diagnosis.

For many women, it's often not until they are navigating the challenges of adulthood—be it through work, motherhood, or shifting social dynamics—that pieces begin to click into place. Untangling the complexities of one's own experience with ADHD can often lead to a harsh awakening, filled with self-reflection and, at times, resentment. Why wasn't I diagnosed sooner? Why was this left unheard? These questions linger, echoing back to those murky days in school when the signs were there, but the recognition was not.

In recognizing the unique female experience of ADHD, we unlock a crucial conversation about how societal frameworks can perpetuate misunderstanding. Women often become experts in masking their symptoms, having spent years learning to navigate a world that demands equanimity. These skills—though they may seem advantageous—often come at a significant emotional cost. Understanding the unique ways ADHD presents in women is the first step in empowering individuals to reclaim their narratives, acknowledging both their struggles and strengths.

Thus, understanding ADHD through the female lens is not merely a diagnostic journey; it is the formulation of a community, a testament to resilience and a reevaluation of success. Women like Sarah and Melissa challenge us to look beyond the surface pain of ADHD manifestations—encouraging us to celebrate creativity, adaptability, and the unique experiences that accompany being a woman with ADHD.

As we proceed through this exploration in the ensuing chapters, we will unravel the complexity of childhood experiences and adult realities, inviting readers to reflect on their lives while illuminating the paths toward understanding, support, and empowerment. Each woman's story serves as a mosaic, painting not merely the struggles but also the beauty of resilience, resourcefulness, and ultimately, growth. The lives affected by ADHD reveal characteristics that are profound, intricate, and distinctly their own—a celebration of the unique female experience in the world of ADHD.

2

Hormonal Influences: The Hormonal Rollercoaster

The journey through life for women with ADHD is akin to riding a rollercoaster, marked by exhilarating highs and daunting drops. This chapter aims to explore the hormonal influences that shape the ADHD experience across key life stages. We will delve into how hormonal fluctuations, from puberty to menopause, intersect with ADHD symptoms, magnifying challenges and providing opportunities for resilience.

The Biological Underpinnings of ADHD and Hormones

At the heart of understanding how hormones impact ADHD is acknowledging the complex interplay between biological and neurological processes. Research indicates that estrogen and progesterone play significant roles in cognitive function and mood regulation, while fluctuations in these hormones can exacerbate ADHD symptoms or trigger new challenges.

During puberty, a significant spike in estrogen occurs, which can amplify both cognitive abilities and ADHD symptoms. For instance, studies suggest that periods of heightened estrogen can enhance verbal skills and memory, potentially masking ADHD traits in girls. As a result, young women may fall prey to the illusion that their ADHD symptoms have diminished, only to resurface more prominently as hormonal levels fluctuate with the menstrual cycle.

Anecdote: Emma's Experience

Emma, a bubbly 24-year-old marketing professional, vividly remembers the disarray of her high school years. She recalls moments when her focus would drift during class discussions, but during those times, she could rely on the heightened energy brought on by positive hormonal shifts. "It was like I had a golden window where I felt invincible," she says. "I would ace my exams without studying too hard because I was just... on fire." However, the veneer would crack each month as PMS crept in, bringing with it distraction, irritability, and cognitive fog.

"During my period, I felt completely overwhelmed," Emma recounts. "It became difficult just to get out of bed. I would misplace things constantly, forget appointments, and feel emotionally volatile." Emma's experience illustrates how hormonal fluctuations can exacerbate the ADHD symptoms that so many women grapple with daily.

Connecting Hormones and Cognitive Function

Contemporary research is beginning to unpack the precise mechanisms behind the relationship between hormonal changes and ADHD symptomatology. One particular study focused on how varying levels of estrogen correlate with attention and cognitive flexibility in women diagnosed with ADHD.

Case Study: Estrogen and Attention Span

In a landmark study involving women diagnosed with ADHD, researchers monitored cognitive performance in relation to menstrual cycle phases. In the follicular phase, when estrogen levels are rising, participants demonstrated notably improved attention spans and working memory. Conversely, during the luteal phase, marked by increased progesterone levels, performance declined, mirroring the heightened ADHD symptoms that many participants reported.

One participant, Anna, remarked, "During the second half of my cycle, I feel like I'm in a fog. I can't concentrate unless there's absolute silence. It's frustrating because I know I'm capable of so much more." This case study illustrates how hormonal cycles are crucial in understanding the ADHD experience and highlights the need for tailored strategies in managing symptoms.

Hormones in Context: Pregnancy and Postpartum

As women move into adulthood, hormonal influences expand beyond monthly cycles. Pregnancy introduces a new array of hormonal fluctuations that can significantly impact ADHD symptoms. Increased estrogen and progesterone can have paradoxical effects; for some women, pregnancy may bring about unexpected focus and calm, while for others, the intensity of the changes may amplify existing ADHD challenges.

Reflections from New Mothers

Nicole, sharing her postpartum experience, recalls, "When I was pregnant, I focused on the changes happening in my body and felt a sense of peace. But once the baby arrived, it was a different reality. I struggled to manage my ADHD symptoms, and the hormonal shifts made it even harder." The postpartum period is notorious for the upheaval it causes in mood and cognitive functioning.

The phenomenon of "baby brain," often jokingly referenced in parenting circles, can feel debilitating for mothers navigating ADHD. Studies indicate that hormonal fluctuations post-birth can affect neurotransmitters like dopamine, often linked to attention and reward processing. Alongside the exhaustion of caring for a newborn, women with ADHD may feel they are fighting an uphill battle.

Menopause: The Final Act of the Hormonal Rollercoaster

As women reach midlife, the hormonal landscape shifts once again with the onset of menopause. The decline in estrogen during this phase can produce myriad cognitive and emotional changes. Women with ADHD may find themselves grappling with an intensification of symptoms like forgetfulness, emotional instability, and increased distractibility.

Shared Experiences and Research Findings

A collaborative study involving women going through menopause assessed changes in ADHD symptom severity in relation to hormonal levels. Remarkably, many women reported that their ADHD symptoms worsened, aligning with significant drops in estrogen during this life stage.

Elaine, a 52-year-old educator, shared, "I thought I was losing my mind. With all the hormonal changes, it was exhausting trying to keep track of my students' names, let alone my own schedule. I felt like I was never going to get through it." Through interviews conducted in the study, it became clear that women navigating this transition experienced similar emotional and cognitive trials, often heightened by the fluctuations in their hormonal levels.

Coping Mechanisms: Finding Balance in the Chaos

While hormonal changes can create formidable challenges, awareness and coping mechanisms can empower women with ADHD. As Emma learned to manage her symptoms during her menstrual cycle, she began tracking her moods and energy levels to prepare for her "low" days. "Understanding my cycle allowed me to create a strategy," she explains. "I started blocking off light work during those times and focused on creative tasks when I felt more energetic."

Establishing routines, maintaining a balanced diet, and engaging in regular physical activity also contribute to stabilizing hormonal levels and improving focus. The concept of self-care becomes especially relevant as women learn to identify their personal cycles and the corresponding challenges they may face.

Reflection and Advocacy

Chapter 2 underscores the importance of recognizing how hormonal disruptions influence the female ADHD experience. The stories of Emma, Anna, Nicole, and Elaine illustrate that awareness is paramount. Each woman's narrative serves as a reminder that, despite the challenges posed by hormonal rollercoasters, understanding and self-compassion are critical tools in navigating ADHD across different life stages.

As more research emerges to highlight the connections between hormones and ADHD, it becomes clear that advocating for personalized treatment options and coping strategies will remain essential. In embracing this journey of awareness, women can transform the tumultuous ride into a path of empowerment, navigating the twists and turns with resilience and strength.

3

The Impacts of ADHD on Relationships

Relationships are fundamental to human experience, woven into the fabric of our lives from childhood through old age. They shape our identities and drive our emotional well-being, yet for many women with ADHD, these connections can be fraught with misunderstandings and challenges tied specifically to the nuances of their condition. In this chapter, we will explore how ADHD can complicate relationships—from friendships to romantic partnerships—by examining communication challenges, emotional dysregulation, and the ways women navigate these interactions. By intertwining anecdotal experiences and case studies, we aim to illuminate the difficulties women face while showcasing strategies for building stronger relationships despite those hurdles.

The Emotional Landscape

At the core of many relationships affected by ADHD lies emotional dysregulation. Women with ADHD may experience intense emotions that can shift rapidly, leaving their partners feeling confused or helpless. This emotional volatility is not solely a product of ADHD itself but may also be exacerbated by societal expectations of women to maintain poise and emotional consistency.

Take Lisa, for example, a 32-year-old freelance graphic designer who has a vivid account of her struggles with friendships. "I often found myself overwhelmed in social situations. If plans changed unexpectedly, I wouldn't just feel disappointed; I'd spiral into deep sadness or anger. I remember my friends thought I was being overly dramatic. They never understood it wasn't just my personality but something more complex. Each time I'd forget a plan or miss a deadline, it felt like I was letting them down, which only intensified my emotional reactions," Lisa reflects.

Her experiences resonate with many women who navigate the tricky waters of friendship while dealing with the impacts of ADHD. The fear of being perceived as unreliable or flaky creates a substantial burden, often leading to withdrawal from social circles. Often, this withdrawal is misinterpreted by friends as disinterest or aloofness, further complicating relationship dynamics.

The Ripple Effect on Romantic Relationships

Romantic partnerships add another layer of complexity for women with ADHD. Communication hiccups, misunderstandings, and differing expectations can lead to recurring conflict. Elena, a 28-year-old software engineer, recounts her first serious relationship: "My partner would often say that I was "tuned out" during conversations. I'd be staring right at him, but my mind was racing, distracted by a million things. It felt like I was failing every time we spoke, and that only made me retreat more. I thought I was being supportive, but I felt invisible, like I had an invisible wall around me."

Research shows that couples affected by ADHD often face unique challenges, such as difficulties in maintaining focus during conversations, managing missed appointments or forgetfulness, and regulating emotional responses. Many times, the non-ADHD partner can feel frustrated or neglected, while the woman with ADHD may feel misunderstood or ashamed. As such, miscommunication becomes a breeding ground for resentment.

In our case study on couples experiencing ADHD's impacts, we follow Allison and Mark, who sought therapy after years of tension in their relationship. Through guided sessions, they began breaking down the barriers that had built up over time. Mark expressed how Allison's tendency to forget things made him feel unimportant: "I would remind her about plans, and when she'd forget, I thought it was because she didn't care. But in therapy, I learned it wasn't that simple."

As they practiced better communication strategies—like using shared calendars and reminders—they found their emotional connection rekindled. This chapter highlights how such therapeutic interventions can promote understanding and empathy, helping couples navigate the complexities of ADHD together.

Insights From Case Studies

In a qualitative study of eighty couples where one partner had ADHD, researchers found that communication strategies significantly impacted relationship satisfaction. Couples who reported using structured communication techniques—like setting aside time for conversations without distractions—found a marked improvement in their emotional health and relationship quality. This emphasizes the importance of proactive measures in fostering healthy interactions.

Figures in the study highlighted that partners who received education about ADHD also exhibited greater patience and understanding, significantly easing tensions. "Learning about my wife's ADHD was a game-changer," noted one partner. "I began to see her challenges not as personal failures, but as realities of her condition, which helped me be more supportive."

Building Emotional Intelligence

One effective strategy for women with ADHD—and their partners—is the cultivation of emotional intelligence. Understanding one's own emotional triggers and responses can drastically improve relational dynamics. Therapy and support groups can provide women an opportunity to explore their feelings and develop coping strategies, enhancing their ability to express themselves clearly and manage reactions.

For instance, Jenna, a 35-year-old who attends an ADHD support group, shared that "learning to articulate my emotions rather than letting them take control has really helped me in my relationships. Instead of lashing out when I feel overwhelmed, I practice explaining my feelings—like, 'I'm annoyed, but I know it's not your fault. Can we talk about this calmly?' This simple shift has eliminated a lot of unnecessary fights."

The Role of Forgiveness

An often overlooked aspect of relationships impacted by ADHD is forgiveness—both self-forgiveness and forgiveness of partners. Many women with ADHD grapple with feelings of guilt about their perceived shortcomings, which can perpetuate a cycle of negativity. Acknowledging past mistakes and moving forward with grace is essential.

Mark's journey with Allison is a notable example of this. After their initial struggles, Mark learned to forgive not just Allison, but himself for the frustrations he had harbored. "I realized holding onto anger for her mistakes wasn't just hurting her; it was hurting me too," he revealed. Reinforcing the idea that forgiveness can pave the way for healing and deeper connections, their bond transformed.

Conclusion

Relationships for women with ADHD are often laden with unique challenges but are also filled with opportunities for growth and understanding. By fostering clear communication, developing emotional intelligence, and embracing forgiveness, women can strengthen their connections with friends and partners alike. Through shared experiences and learned strategies, these relationships can evolve from misunderstandings into powerful, supportive alliances that celebrate the unique strengths women with ADHD bring to the table.

As this chapter illustrates, the road to strong relationships may be winding, but it is one that offers rich rewards—a sense of belonging, love, and mutual support that can enhance the experience of life with ADHD. In the following chapters, we will explore how these interpersonal dynamics transition into career challenges and triumphs, highlighting the diverse implications of ADHD throughout various life stages.

4

Career Challenges and Triumphs for Women with ADHD

Navigating the professional landscape can often feel like an overwhelming obstacle course, especially for women with Attention Deficit Hyperactivity Disorder (ADHD). The intricacies of workplace dynamics, combined with the unique symptoms of ADHD—such as difficulties in organization, time management, emotional regulation, and impulse control—create challenges that can hinder career advancement. However, the reality also includes tales of triumph, adaptability, and strength among women who have learned to navigate these waters. This chapter explores these realities, providing a lens into the professional lives of women with ADHD through anecdotes and case studies.

Struggles in the Workplace

Consider Rachel, a project manager in her thirties who shared her journey through professional burnout. Rachel had always been passionate about her work, excelling in creative aspects and strategic planning. However, as her responsibilities grew, so did the expectations placed upon her, both by herself and her colleagues.

"I always felt like I had to prove myself," Rachel explains. "But juggling multiple tasks while keeping track of deadlines became overwhelming. I would forget meetings or misplace important documents, and then the anxiety would spiral." Rachel's tale is a common story among women with ADHD; where their creativity and determination often become overshadowed by the challenges posed by their symptoms.

Rachel reached a breaking point when she found herself working late nights, struggling to keep up, and starting to fall behind on projects. Recognizing the toll this was taking on her mental health, she sought help. After discussing her symptoms with a mental health professional, she gained insights into how ADHD influenced her work style. This realization served as a turning point.

"I'm not 'bad' at my job. I just needed to explore ways to work with my brain, not against it," Rachel said. With her therapist's guidance, she requested accommodations at work—such as more structured project timelines, the use of digital reminders, and the ability to focus on one task at a time for set periods.

Redefining Success

Rachel's experience shows that success in a career for women with ADHD doesn't necessarily look like a straight trajectory upward. It often involves taking the time to redefine what success means alongside acknowledgment of personal limits and unique strengths.

To illustrate this concept further, consider a longitudinal study examining women with ADHD across various professions. Participants ranged from educators to corporate executives and creative entrepreneurs. Each participant disclosed not only the barriers they faced—such as discrimination, gender bias, and ADHD stigma—but also the coping strategies that enabled them to thrive.

The study revealed a recurring theme: successful women with ADHD often found innovative ways to align their work environments with their strengths. Many opted for flexible job roles that allowed for a high degree of autonomy, which is crucial for managing attention variability. Others pursued careers that catered to their strong creative skills or those that involved rapid problem-solving.

For instance, one participant, a graphic designer named Laura, recounted how she leveraged her ADHD to excel in her job. "When I'm in the zone, I can hyper-focus on a project like nobody else. It's like the world fades away and all my thoughts coalesce into a single idea. I've learned to capitalize on those moments." Laura learned to structure her work schedule to include blocks of time specifically set aside for deep-focus creative tasks and combined them with regular breaks, which kept her energized and productive.

Shifting Perspectives on ADHD in the Workplace

The workplace experiences of women with ADHD also underline the need for a shift in perspective surrounding ADHD's impact. For many women, the traditional work environment is not built to accommodate the needs that arise from diverse attention profiles. The stigma of traditional office expectations often adds to feelings of inadequacy and frustration.

It's essential for workplaces to recognize the value of neurodiversity. Employers are increasingly more aware of how diverse working styles can enrich organizational culture. Yet, there remains a gap in training and awareness for leadership and

HR professionals about how best to support employees with ADHD. This is where communal dialogue and advocacy play a fundamental role.

The case study of a tech company that instituted a tailored approach to workplace accommodations exemplifies this. By implementing policies that supported flexible work schedules, providing organizational tools, and facilitating open discussions about ADHD and its impact, the company saw notable improvements in productivity and employee satisfaction, particularly among neurodivergent staff. Employees were encouraged to engage with their managers about their individual needs, fostering an environment of understanding and inclusivity.

Embracing Creative Strengths

Beyond coping strategies and accommodations, many women find empowerment in embracing the unique aspects of their thinking that ADHD brings. Creativity often emerges as a strength among those with ADHD. The women in the longitudinal study often noted that their divergent thinking patterns enabled them to solve problems in innovative ways, generating fresh ideas that stood out in the workplace.

One particularly compelling case was that of Kamala, an entrepreneur who founded a small business that centers around eco-friendly fashion. Kamala explained, "I think differently, and that's my superpower. I connect dots that others don't see and draw inspiration from unexpected places." Her account is a testament to the multifaceted capabilities of women with ADHD who navigate their careers while harnessing their strengths.

By viewing ADHD through a lens of potential rather than limitation, Kamala embodies the spirit of resilience that many women cultivate in the face of challenges. She networks with other women who share similar experiences, forming a support group that further amplifies their artistic endeavors and encourages professional collaborations.

The Path Forward

Navigating a career with ADHD presents distinct challenges, yet it is not solely defined by struggle. Women like Rachel, Laura, and Kamala exemplify the hopeful journeys of learning to balance their professional lives while embracing their unique ways of thinking. The workforce can benefit from diversity in neurodivergent perspective, leading to innovative ideas and dynamic solutions.

As we conclude this chapter, it is important to reinforce the message that women with ADHD possess extraordinary gifts that when nurtured can lead to remarkable professional achievements. Empowering themselves with knowledge, seeking accommodations, and embracing their creativity, they turn challenges into pathways for growth and advocacy in workplaces. Through their narratives, women with ADHD inspire others, demonstrating that struggles can indeed lead to triumphs in the various stages of a fulfilling career. Their journeys remind us that understanding, support, and self-advocacy are essential ingredients in transforming the challenges of living with ADHD into opportunities for success.

5

Self-Advocacy: Navigating Diagnosis and Treatment

The journey of obtaining a diagnosis and managing treatment for ADHD can be a complicated path, especially for women. Self-advocacy is crucial, serving as the bridge between personal experiences and professional guidance. This chapter dives deep into the concept of self-advocacy, illustrating its monumental importance in the lives of women with ADHD. Through narratives and case studies, we will explore how women can navigate the often overwhelming healthcare system to articulate their needs, motivating them to seek appropriate diagnoses and treatment options.

The Importance of Self-Advocacy

Self-advocacy in the context of ADHD means understanding one's own symptoms, being able to communicate these symptoms clearly, and knowing your rights as a patient. For many women, however, societal expectations and stigmas surrounding mental health can obstruct this process. The notion that one must not appear 'difficult' or insist on special treatments can create an environment where women feel they must downplay their struggles.

Maria, a 35-year-old mother of two, exemplifies this struggle. Maria had struggled with disorganization and procrastination throughout her adult life but often attributed these issues to being a busy mother. After years of feeling misunderstood by her healthcare providers, Maria finally found the courage to articulate her concerns. "It was hard," she admits. "I felt that I needed to justify my experiences because I didn't fit the typical mold of someone with ADHD. I worried they'd think I was just lazy or overwhelmed as any mother would be."

Maria's story illustrates the inner turmoil that many women face. Often taught to value accommodation for others above their own needs, they may sacrifice their voices in healthcare settings where they should be firmly and unambiguously represented.

The Road to Diagnosis

Many women experience lengthy and convoluted journeys to obtain a formal ADHD diagnosis. The symptoms of ADHD often manifest differently in women compared to men, leading some practitioners to misattribute their struggles as resulting from anxiety, depression, or other co-occurring conditions. This minimizes the urgency of their plight.

Consider the case of Laura, who, after years of battling with feelings of inadequacy, visited numerous doctors and therapists. Each appointment ended in mixed signals—while some practitioners dismissed her complaints, others proposed alternative diagnoses that felt wrong. It was only after an eventual referral to a specialist that Laura finally received her ADHD diagnosis, which felt like both a relief and an additional burden.

"Until I got that diagnosis, it was like I was walking around in a fog. I knew something was off, but I couldn't pinpoint what it was," Laura recounts. "Getting that diagnosis was both liberating and terrifying. It named my struggles, and I could finally start to learn how to navigate them."

Laura's experience is not unique but rather a common narrative among women seeking to make sense of their lives as they face unrecognized or misdiagnosed ADHD symptoms. The challenge is not just in receiving a diagnosis but in knowing how to ask the right questions during consultations and persistently advocating for their own mental health.

Communication Strategies

Effective communication with healthcare providers is vital for self-advocacy. To begin, women should prepare to discuss their experiences comprehensively. This can involve taking notes before appointments, outlining symptoms, or bringing along the insights of trusted family members or friends. Women like Maria found that using specific language regarding their symptoms often helped: Instead of just stating that they felt "scattered," they articulated examples—like forgetting appointments or feeling overwhelmingly emotional.

Additionally, women can benefit from understanding their rights as patients. Knowing the legalities surrounding diagnosis and treatment in their location empowers women to raise concerns about both their mental and physical health. It also helps diminish feelings of inadequacy or guilt associated with seeking help.

An effective strategy employed by Maria was to keep a daily journal documenting her symptoms, challenges, and triumphs.

"Having my experiences written down made them real in a way," she explains. "When I shared my journal entries with my therapist, it became a tangible expression of what I was going through."

Case Study: Diverse Treatment Paths

Two women from distinctly different backgrounds, Sophia and Rachel, showcase how self-advocacy can shape individual treatment journeys.

Sophia, a successful corporate attorney in her 40s, initially felt paralyzed by her ADHD symptoms. Her struggle with focus and organization led to severe anxiety, causing her professional life to falter. After a long period of frustration, she took matters into her own hands, researching potential treatments and advocating for her needs at work. Eventually, she was able to negotiate accommodations that allowed her to excel in her role while managing her ADHD. She highlights how important it was to present a well-researched case to her supervisor. "I brought printouts and studies about ADHD in the workplace," she recalls with pride. "I needed to make it clear that my needs were not just personal inconveniences but well-documented aspects of ADHD."

Conversely, Rachel's journey had a different flavor of self-advocacy. She opted for a holistic approach to treatment after her diagnosis, engaging with various wellness practitioners along with traditional medication. She joined community circles focused on mindfulness and self-care practices, translating her experience into a rich tapestry of personal tools. This proactive step required her to engage with multiple specialists—nutritionists, yoga instructors, and life coaches—tailoring her treatment to complement her ADHD symptoms.

Both women's stories illustrate the role of self-advocacy in shaping treatment factors. Whether it is through a professional lens or a more holistic approach, both paths exemplify taking charge of one's health and showcasing a refusal to be dismissed.

The Emotional Toll

Despite the determination to advocate for themselves, many women face emotional tolls during this process. The fatigue from advocating and navigating complex healthcare landscapes can leave them feeling overwhelmed. The weight of societal expectations often adds layers to this burden, creating additional stress. The journey may feel Sisyphean: just when they feel they've made progress, new barriers or challenges arise.

Maria's journey encapsulates this exhaustion. "There were days I felt like an imposter in my own life. Just when I thought I had the tools to manage, something new would pop up," she reflects. This emotional labor can lead to burnout if women do not prioritize their mental health alongside their advocacy work. Thus, self-care becomes an essential component of self-advocacy.

Conclusion

Self-advocacy is, ultimately, a critical skill for women navigating the ADHD landscape. Through effective communication, preparation, and an understanding of one's rights, women can work to ensure their experiences are validated and addressed. Maria, Laura, Sophia, and Rachel exemplify how the power of self-advocacy not only fosters a deeper understanding of their ADHD but also propels them toward appropriate treatment options.

As we progress through life with ADHD, embracing the act

of self-advocacy can lead to empowerment. It transforms the internal struggles into external dialogues, nurturing an environment where women can thrive rather than merely survive. In the quest for mental wellness, understanding the art of advocacy is not just beneficial—it is essential. In the subsequent chapters, we will explore mindfulness and coping strategies which complement this indispensable skill, providing further tools for navigating the complexities of the ADHD experience.

6

Mindfulness and Coping Strategies

In the ever-evolving landscape of managing ADHD, mindfulness emerges as a pivotal tool, guiding women to navigate their unique challenges with grace and self-awareness. This chapter delves deeply into the art and science of mindfulness, exploring its profound impact on women living with ADHD. We'll look at compelling anecdotes from remarkable women who have embarked on this journey of self-discovery, as well as a detailed case study on community workshops designed to facilitate mindfulness and coping strategies.

The Power of Mindfulness

Mindfulness transcends mere relaxation techniques; it is an empowering practice grounded in the present moment, fostering a profound awareness of thoughts, feelings, and bodily sensations. For women with ADHD, the practice of mindfulness can serve as a lifeline, offering strategies to combat the distractions and emotional turbulence that often accompany the condition.

Jenna's Journey

Take Jenna, a 35-year-old graphic designer who struggled with maintaining focus amidst a chaotic work environment. Her ADHD manifested in pervasive distractibility and intense bouts of anxiety that often left her overwhelmed. After learning about mindfulness through an online article, she decided to give meditation a try. Initially skeptical, Jenna committed to a 10-minute daily practice of mindfulness meditation.

After several weeks, the transformation began. "At first, it was hard to sit still," she recalls. "My mind raced with a thousand thoughts: what to eat for lunch, overdue emails, and plans for the weekend. But eventually, I learned to gently redirect my thoughts back to my breath." Over time, Jenna found that these moments of pause not only improved her focus but also reduced her anxiety dramatically.

Mindfulness provided Jenna with a new toolkit. When she noticed her mind wandering, Jenna learned to acknowledge the distractions without judgment, allowing herself to return to her tasks with renewed clarity. This simple practice fostered a sense of ease in her day-to-day life. The riddles of ADHD no longer felt insurmountable, but rather, manageable challenges she could approach with awareness.

Mindfulness Techniques for Coping

As Jenna's story illustrates, mindfulness techniques can serve as powerful coping mechanisms for women with ADHD. Here, we explore a selection of practical exercises, each designed to enhance focus, reduce anxiety, and cultivate emotional regulation.

1. **Breathing Exercises**: Simple breathing techniques are foundational to mindfulness. One effective exercise is the "4-7-8 Breath" where one inhales for four counts, holds the breath for seven counts, and exhales for eight counts. This process can ground the practitioner, reducing anxiety and increasing attentiveness.
2. **Body Scan Meditation**: This involves focusing attention on different parts of the body, from the head to the toes. As one notices sensations—such as tension or relaxation—this technique helps cultivate a connection between mind and body, enhancing self-awareness.
3. **Mindful Journaling**: Writing thoughts and feelings down in a journal can help create clarity. A journaling technique called "stream of consciousness" allows individuals to write without restrictions for a set time, freeing the mind from clutter and revealing deeper insights.
4. **Mindful Walking**: Incorporating mindfulness into simple activities, such as walking, can turn a mundane task into a meditative practice. Paying attention to each step, the sensations of the ground underfoot, and the rhythm of breathing transforms these moments into opportunities for grounding.
5. **Gratitude Practice**: Taking time daily or weekly to reflect on what one is grateful for can shift focus from negative thought patterns towards positivity—an essential practice for emotional regulation, especially in individuals with ADHD.

Case Study: Community Workshop Series

To further illuminate the transformative power of mindfulness, we turn to a community workshop series designed to teach coping strategies to women with ADHD. Conducted over six weeks, the workshops were attended by a diverse group of twenty women, ranging from teenagers to professionals in their thirties.

Workshop Structure: Each session included guided mindfulness practices, discussions on ADHD-related challenges, and sharing of personal experiences. Participants engaged in breathing exercises, group meditations, and mindful movement sessions, providing a supportive environment for learning and growth.

Measurable Improvements: To gauge the workshop's efficacy, participants completed pre- and post-workshop assessments measuring attention spans, anxiety levels, and overall well-being. Remarkably, the data indicated that 80% of participants reported a decrease in anxiety levels, while 75% noted improvements in their ability to focus during tasks.

Particularly impactful was the shared experience of women discussing their unique challenges, emphasizing the role a supportive community plays in managing ADHD. As one participant noted, "I never realized how much I needed to connect with others like me. Sharing our struggles was therapeutic."

Through these workshops, participants not only learned practical mindfulness techniques but also discovered the importance of community in their ADHD journey. The feedback emphasized how creating a space where women could openly share experiences helped dismantle stigma and fostered resilience, illustrating that mindfulness extends beyond individual practice into a collective, transformative experience.

The Future of Mindfulness in Managing ADHD

As we reflect on the experiences shared by Jenna and participants of the workshop series, a compelling narrative emerges: mindfulness is not simply a set of techniques; it is an evolving, adaptable practice that can be tailored to the needs of women with ADHD at various life stages.

Adopting mindfulness can become an integral part of managing ADHD, not only enhancing coping strategies but also enabling women to embrace their unique experiences holistically. As they immerse themselves in mindfulness, they find greater emotional balance, improved focus, and a deeper understanding of themselves.

In the following chapters, we will explore how these skills intertwine with body image, societal pressures, and various life stages, highlighting the broader implications of living with ADHD. By recognizing the intersection of these experiences, we can begin to cultivate a more nuanced understanding of the ADHD journey for women—a journey enriched by the practices of mindfulness and community support.

7

Body Image, ADHD & Societal Pressures

The intersection of body image, self-esteem, and Attention Deficit Hyperactivity Disorder (ADHD) is a complex and often troubled terrain for many women. In a society that perpetuates narrow definitions of beauty and success, women with ADHD face unique challenges that not only affect their mental health but also their relationships with their bodies. This chapter explores these challenges through personal anecdotes and case studies, highlighting the struggle against societal pressures and the impulsivity often associated with ADHD.

To illustrate this struggle, we will delve into the experiences of several women as they navigate the tumultuous waters of body image while grappling with ADHD.

Tasha's Journey: Impulsivity and Body Image

Tasha, a 32-year-old graphic designer, recalls the moment she realized her self-image was intricately tied to her ADHD. "I've always been drawn to food. It provides comfort, a momentary escape from the chaos in my mind," she reflects. But this impulsive behavior has often led her to binge eat, showcasing a food relationship complicated by ADHD.

Tasha's backstory is not uncommon. Women with ADHD often struggle with impulse control, which can manifest in eating habits that deviate from societal expectations of moderation and fitness. This impulsivity is exacerbated by powerful media portrayals of the "ideal body," leaving many women like Tasha feeling inadequate. "Every time I look in the mirror, all I see are the things that don't fit with the ideals. It feels like I'm fighting a battle I can't win," she admits.

Throughout her life, Tasha faced bullying and criticism for her weight. During her teenage years, the relentless media images of ultra-thin models and socially constructed standards of beauty cemented a negative self-image in her mind. "When I was a teen, I wanted to fit in so badly that I would try every diet that came my way. I'd follow them for a few days, maybe weeks, and then I'd just crash and revert to old habits," she explains. Each crash left her feeling more defeated, reinforcing the cycle of body dissatisfaction and emotional distress.

Case Study: Focus Groups on Women's Perception of Beauty

In a recent research initiative, focus groups were conducted with women diagnosed with ADHD to better understand how societal expectations shape their perceptions of body image. Participants reported a shared sentiment: the weight of expectations often overshadowed their accomplishments and strengths. In discussions, many women shared Tasha's experiences, noting that their ADHD sometimes exacerbated feelings of worthlessness connected to their body image.

One participant, Sarah, articulated a common struggle: "It's like my brain is saying, 'You're not good enough because you don't look like her,' yet I know I'm doing amazing things at work and in my personal life. The disconnect is maddening." This cognitive dissonance is a hallmark of the ADHD experience, often leading to emotional dysregulation. Many women described how societal standards of beauty affected their self-esteem, correlating directly with their ADHD symptoms, including anxiety and depression.

The findings from these focus groups underscore the profound impact that societal beauty standards have on women with ADHD. Participants expressed longing for a world where diverse body types are celebrated rather than vilified, revealing how acceptance could lead to enhanced mental well-being. "If only we could redefine what 'beautiful' means to include all shapes and sizes, maybe then we could all feel like we belong," said one participant.

Impacts of Societal Pressures on Mental Health

The societal pressures that accompany body image concern often lead to more complex issues for women with ADHD. The emotional regulation difficulties associated with ADHD can amplify negative feelings about oneself. When societal standards dictate perfection, the struggle becomes twofold: wrestling with the impulsivity of ADHD while simultaneously dealing with the self-imposed pressures of an unattainable body image.

Women with ADHD may find themselves caught in a cycle: impulsively indulging in food as a means of comfort during emotionally taxing moments, only to feel guilty afterward due to societal judgments. This vicious cycle was captured in the case study where participants noted that ADHD behaviors such as forgetfulness and inattention often extend to self-care routines, impacting exercise and diet maintenance.

This reality often leads to heightened anxiety and depression, as Tasha articulated, "Every time I feel like I'm making progress, I see an Instagram post or magazine cover that reinforces how far from 'perfect' I am." Such interactions are a reminder that society's ideals can often be toxic, especially for those already struggling with their mental health.

Strategies for Navigating Body Image

Addressing body image issues in women with ADHD requires a multi-faceted approach. It's crucial to cultivate a supportive environment where diverse body types are celebrated and where women understand that their worth isn't contingent upon their appearance.

One effective strategy emerged from the focus group discussions: creating supportive communities where women can share their experiences without the weight of societal judgment. Tasha, inspired by her newfound sense of community, began organizing workshops that encourage body positivity among women with ADHD. "We created a space where we can talk about our struggles, but also celebrate the things we love about ourselves. It's empowering," she says.

Another strategy involves mindfulness and self-compassion techniques to help mitigate negative self-talk. Tasha emphasizes, "Learning how to talk to myself compassionately has been life-changing. I still have a long way to go, but I'm no longer my harshest critic." Integrating consistent mindfulness practices has proven to help many women navigate their emotional responses better.

Conclusion: Reclaiming Body Image Amid ADHD

Ultimately, body image is a deeply personal experience that

interweaves with ADHD in complex ways. For women like Tasha, reclaiming the narrative means acknowledging both their struggles and strengths. The journey of overcoming societal pressures is ongoing, but the power of community, self-advocacy, and mindfulness equips women to navigate this landscape with greater resilience.

As conversations around body image evolve, it becomes increasingly vital to recognize and support those who live with ADHD, championing their right to feel confident in their own skin, regardless of societal pressures. The journey towards embracing one's body, shaped by unique ADHD experiences, is not just a personal endeavor but a collective movement towards acceptance and celebration of diversity in all its forms.

8

Transitions and Life Stages: From Adolescence to Adulthood

Navigating life's transitions can be daunting for anyone, but for women with Attention-Deficit/Hyperactivity Disorder (ADHD), these turning points can evoke unique challenges. Adolescence is often marked by intense self-discovery and social pressures, while young adulthood introduces expectations around independence, careers, and relationships. Motherhood, both thrilling and overwhelming, adds yet another layer of complexity to the ADHD experience. In this chapter, we will explore the multifaceted difficulties faced by women with ADHD as they traverse these critical life stages, drawing from personal anecdotes and comprehensive case studies to illustrate the intricate interplay between ADHD and life transitions.

Childhood to Adolescence: The Formative Years

The transition from childhood to adolescence is rarely smooth. For women with ADHD, compounded societal expectations can create a perfect storm of confusion and self-doubt. Nicole, a 26-year-old mother, recalls walking the tightrope of adolescence with ADHD. "I always felt behind my peers," she recalls. "While they were getting their driver's licenses or planning for college, I was still struggling to remember my homework or keep track of my friends' names."

Nicole's experiences were often complicated by emotional dysregulation, a common symptom of ADHD in females. She remembers feeling a sense of isolation as friendships toppled due to forgetfulness and impulsivity: "My friends would invite me to events, but I would forget about them or lose track of time. I started to withdraw because I didn't want to deal with the awkwardness."

As we explore Nicole's journey, it becomes clear that many young women experience the same feeling of being adrift in a sea of expectations. It is a sentiment echoed in case studies focusing on female adolescents diagnosed with ADHD—a group often overlooked in traditional ADHD research. These studies reveal that, unlike their male counterparts, girls frequently exhibit internalizing symptoms like anxiety and low self-esteem, leading to higher rates of emotional disorders and lesser acknowledgment of ADHD symptoms.

Young Adulthood: Pathways to Independence

As females with ADHD transition into young adulthood, they face increased pressure to gain independence, pursue higher education, and build careers while dealing with the challenges inherent to their condition. Nicole's story takes an illuminating turn in her early twenties when she began to navigate these realms. "College was a disaster," she admits, recalling late-night cramming, forgotten assignments, and widespread procrastination. "I felt lost in the shuffle and overwhelmed by the workload."

Research studies indicate that women with ADHD often use executive function skills inadequately, leading to difficulties in academic environments. Many struggle with organization and time management, making higher education an uphill battle. These challenges are magnified by social pressures to appear competent and composed—expectations that can feel insurmountable for those who constantly fight against the tide of ADHD symptoms.

Ultimately, Nicole made the decision to seek help. After an emotional moment of reckoning, she reached out to a counseling service on campus, where she was first introduced to coping strategies aimed at women with ADHD. The therapy not only equipped her with tools for focusing but also initiated a process of acceptance: "For the first time, I felt like I wasn't alone in this struggle. I started connecting with other girls who were experiencing similar frustrations."

Motherhood: A New Chapter of Challenges

Transitioning into motherhood adds yet another layer of complexity to a woman with ADHD's life experience. The demands of pregnancy, childbirth, and parenting require a level of organization and attentiveness that can overwhelm even the most capable individuals. Nicole's story continues as she faces motherhood, which brings both joy and guilt. "I felt elated to be a new mom, but there were days when my ADHD felt crippling," she shares.

She describes the chaos of managing an infant's schedule alongside her own struggles to maintain routine: "I'd forget to feed myself while keeping track of feeding, diaper changes, and nap times for my daughter. The guilt would spiral; I thought, 'How can I be a good mom if I can't even manage my own routine?'"

Nicole's experiences resonate with findings from various studies on women with ADHD who become mothers. These studies often highlight the cognitive load and emotional strain that accompany parenting, especially the pressures placed on women to balance domestic responsibilities, careers, and personal well-being. Many report feeling overwhelmed, leading to a cycle where feelings of inadequacy trigger ADHD symptoms, which in turn exacerbate feelings of guilt and frustration.

Adapting Strategies for Life Transitions

Transforming these daunting challenges into manageable experiences involves adopting practical strategies. For Nicole, this included establishing a support network. She became active in a local mother's group of women with ADHD, where sharing stories and strategies became a salve for her worries. "Talking to other moms was liberating," she notes. "We talked about our struggles—forgetting appointments, losing track of toys, and emotional meltdowns. It helped reduce the isolation I felt and offered practical solutions."

Research supports the effectiveness of peer support networks for women with ADHD, as they can provide emotional backing and actionable strategies for navigating challenging transitions. Elements of group therapy sessions that emphasize shared experiences and active problem-solving can significantly improve mood and coping skills among participants.

Recognizing Progress and Strengths

As women with ADHD traverse these life stages, it is crucial to acknowledge the strengths that emerge from their experiences. Nicole demonstrates resilience as she adapts her approaches to meet changing demands: "I learned to rely on my planner religiously, and I use reminders on my phone for both my appointments and my daughter's," she explains. "I've reframed my mindset; instead of seeing my ADHD as a liability, I recognize how it has pushed me to be creative in finding solutions."

The case studies reviewed throughout this chapter highlight similar resilience among women learning to navigate life's stages with ADHD. Many have transformed the challenges into sources of strength, developing exceptional coping mechanisms characterized by adaptability, creativity, and fierce determination.

Looking Ahead: Embracing Transitions

As this chapter highlights, navigating life's transitions with ADHD is not a linear journey but a series of evolving landscapes filled with hurdles and triumphs. By amplifying their voices and experiences, women like Nicole share their struggles and victories, offering hope and solidarity for others walking similar paths.

As women with ADHD continue to adapt through the transitions of adolescence, young adulthood, and motherhood, they prove that beyond the chaos, there is the possibility of connection, understanding, and ultimately, empowerment. The strategies they develop become a toolkit for resilience that can be passed down through generations, shaping future narratives of ADHD not merely as challenges but as springboards for growth and transformation.

9

Community Support: Building a Network

In the intricate landscape of ADHD, where the personal experience often feels isolating, the value of community support cannot be overstated. For many women navigating the turbulent waters of ADHD, finding a network of understanding and acceptance can be transformative. This chapter will explore how communal ties—whether through in-person support groups, online forums, or social networks—can enhance coping mechanisms, foster resilience, and ultimately enrich the quality of life for women with ADHD.

The Search for Connection

Angela, a 34-year-old freelance graphic designer, felt isolated in her struggles with ADHD until she stumbled upon an online forum designed specifically for women with the condition. Like many, she had long been battling feelings of inadequacy and confusion stemming from the chaotic world of her mind. While others seemed to glide through life effortlessly, Angela often found herself overwhelmed by the minutiae of daily tasks—

organization remained a distant dream, and time management felt like an elusive art form.

However, upon joining the online community, Angela was greeted with stories strikingly similar to her own. Shared experiences of forgetfulness, emotional dysregulation, and anxiety struck a chord. For the first time, she felt a deep sense of validation. The connection she formed with other women who understood the nuances of living with ADHD provided her with solace and perspective. "It's like suddenly being part of a club," Angela recounted. "A club that no one wants to join, but once you're in, you realize you're not alone."

The Power of Shared Experiences

The essence of community support lies in shared experiences, which can alleviate feelings of isolation. For many women, simply having a safe space to talk about the intricacies of their ADHD can lead to revelations that foster healing and self-acceptance. Peer support groups, both in person and online, facilitate spaces where women can be unfiltered and honest about their struggles, victories, and everything in between.

Case in point, a local support group in a medium-sized city highlighted these dynamics beautifully. The group, consisting of ten women ranging from their twenties to their fifties, gathered weekly to share struggles and celebrate victories. Many reported experiencing improvements in mood simply by attending these meetings. The women conducted activities such as brainstorming organization tips, playing games designed to enhance focus, and engaging in mindfulness exercises together.

In one particular session, they decided to share their stories of ADHD-related setbacks. Sally, a mother of two, recounted her latest struggle with time management, describing an instance when she misread her schedule, leading to her missing an important parent-teacher meeting. Instead of shame, however, the group responded with empathy and laughter, sharing similar incidents they had endured. The collective acknowledgment fostered a supportive atmosphere where vulnerability was met with compassion, converting moments of self-doubt into learning experiences.

Online Communities: Breaking Geographical Barriers

While in-person support groups play a crucial role, online platforms have transformed the landscape of ADHD support. Angela's experience highlights the unique benefits of these digital spaces. They transcend geographical limitations, allowing women from diverse backgrounds to connect and share their stories, advice, and coping strategies.

Research has shown that online communities can significantly enhance feelings of acceptance and connectedness among women with ADHD. In studies focused on mental health support groups, participants reported higher levels of self-esteem and decreased feelings of isolation when engaging in online forums. The anonymity provided by the internet can also empower women to express thoughts they may feel uncomfortable sharing in person.

Furthermore, digital spaces foster a form of support that is particularly comforting for those with ADHD; the ability to connect asynchronously allows for thoughtful engagement. Women can return to discussions at their convenience, ensuring they can process information without the pressure of real-time interaction.

Angela mentioned a particular thread about the intersection of ADHD and entrepreneurship that transformed her professional life. Voices in the thread included women managing businesses, sharing strategies for keeping organized while ensuring creativity flowed. These connections not only helped Angela thrive in her work but also inspired her to reframe her ADHD traits as assets.

The Role of Mentorship and Leadership in Community Building

A critical aspect of community support is the mentorship that often arises within these networks. Mentors can provide guidance and encouragement to those navigating their ADHD diagnosis, especially younger women or those newly diagnosed.

Sophia's role as a mentor in her local ADHD women's group showcases the significant impact mentorship can have. Having been diagnosed as a teenager, she struggled for years before finally learning to harness her ADHD traits into strengths. In her role as a mentor, she emphasized the importance of resilience, goal-setting, and the practical application of coping strategies.

During meetings, she would lead discussions on developing personalized ADHD management techniques or stress management, drawing from her experiences. "I want others to see that ADHD doesn't define you; it can be a powerful tool if you learn to leverage it," Sophia reiterated. Her guidance inspired many of the group's younger members to pursue their goals confidently, creating a virtuous cycle of empowerment and support.

Measuring the Impact of Support Networks

The outcomes from participating in support networks often speak for themselves. By participating in a local support group, community members reported increased self-esteem, improved coping mechanisms, and reduced symptoms of anxiety.

An informal study conducted by facilitators of the group

evaluated participants' emotional and mental health before and after attending the support group over a six-month period. Results indicated a marked improvement in overall mood and coping skills among the participants, demonstrating the tangible positive impact of community support on mental health.

Creating Your Own Support Network

For those who may not yet be part of a community, taking the first step towards building connections can be daunting. One effective approach is to look for local ADHD support groups through hospitals, community centers, or university health services. Online platforms, such as Facebook groups or forums dedicated to ADHD, can also serve as accessible entry points.

Remember that building a community is an ongoing process; it thrives on openness, sharing, and mutual respect. Starting small can lead to substantial rewards, as connections deepen over time.

Engagement in a community can serve as a lifeline, transforming challenges related to ADHD into shared experiences that foster solidarity, resilience, and empowerment. Women navigating ADHD don't have to do so in solitude; together, they can build supportive networks that celebrate their unique strengths and communal understanding.

Conclusion

Building community support is not merely about finding allies; it's about creating a transformative environment where women with ADHD can thrive. As Angela found her way into the folds of her supportive online community, so too can others encounter their networks of understanding and empowerment. As advocates for each other, women can rise above their challenges and embrace the rich tapestry of their lives shaped by ADHD. In this bond, they find not only recognition but strength, turning obstacles into milestones and collective experiences into growth. Together, they are not just managing ADHD; they are defining what it means to live powerfully with it.

10

Embracing Your ADHD Superpowers

As the sun dipped below the skyline, casting a warm golden hue across the city, Sophie sat at her desk, surrounded by colorful sketches and half-finished projects. The aroma of brewed coffee wafted through her small studio apartment, mingling with the scent of the fresh paint drying on the canvases. With a contagious energy that seemed to radiate from her being, she reflected on her journey as a woman with ADHD. Today, she felt a sense of empowerment that had eluded her in her early years, and she was eager to share her story.

ADHD has often been framed as a limitation, a label that can feel heavy and burdensome. Yet, for many women like Sophie, it can also be a source of unique strengths. Creativity, resilience, and hyper-focus are three remarkable traits that can emerge from the ADHD experience. This chapter explores how women can embrace these so-called "superpowers" and transform ADHD into a tool for personal and professional achievement.

The Journey of Self-Acceptance
From an early age, Sophie often felt out of sync with her

peers. In the classroom, while others seemed to absorb lessons with ease, she grappled with disorganization and distractibility. Teachers labeled her as daydreaming, a term that made her feel invisible—a mere speck in a sea of structured desks and ordered minds. It wasn't until her late twenties, after finally seeking a diagnosis, that she began to untangle the complex interplay between her creativity and her ADHD.

"I used to think that my brain was just wired differently in a bad way," Sophie recalled, her voice a mixture of nostalgia and triumph. "But once I learned about ADHD, I started to see these traits as gifts. My hyper-focus, for example, allows me to dive deep into my art for hours on end. I can create something incredibly intricate and detailed, often losing myself completely in the process. It's exhilarating."

Sophie's experience is not an anomaly. Many women with ADHD discover that their unique way of thinking often leads to exceptional creative potential. Case studies have shown that individuals with ADHD frequently thrive in environments that require innovation and out-of-the-box thinking. From artists to entrepreneurs, those who harness their ADHD traits can create powerful and meaningful work.

Celebrating Creativity

Numerous stories echo Sophie's journey into embracing creativity as a superpower. For instance, Jenna—a graphic designer—found that her impulsivity often translated into spontaneous ideas. In a brainstorming session that would typically exhaust others, Jenna would be energizing the room with new concepts and designs. She learned to overcome her moments of doubt by viewing her impulsive bursts of inspiration as essential part of her creative process.

The importance of celebrating creativity cannot be understated. A study conducted in collaboration with several ADHD coaching organizations revealed that women who engaged in creative outlets reported higher levels of self-esteem and fulfillment. These women were encouraged to pursue their passions without the fear of judgment—a vital component to harnessing ADHD strengths.

Embracing creativity has its challenges; the chaotic nature of ADHD can sometimes lead to unfinished projects. Yet, Sophie learned to navigate this through organization strategies compatible with her ADHD style. Embracing digital tools such as project management apps, she was able to break her creative processes into manageable tasks, allowing room for both spontaneity and structure.

Resilience: The Heart of the ADHD Experience

Resilience is another hallmark of the ADHD experience. Overcoming challenges and navigating a world that often overlooks the experiences of women with ADHD requires an inherent strength. A poignant case study focused on a group of women entrepreneurs revealed that their struggles with ADHD provided them with an acute ability to pivot in the face of adversity.

"Every setback felt like a lesson in disguise," said Lisa, one of the entrepreneurs featured in the study. "Having ADHD taught me to adapt quickly, which is a crucial skill when running a business. The ability to think on my feet? It's essential when everything seems to change in an instant."

Women like Sophie and Lisa often find that their journeys of resilience are intertwined with their capacity to connect with others. By sharing their stories and struggles, they not only empower themselves but also create a network of strength for others. This reciprocal relationship enhances community ties, fostering a culture of encouragement and shared triumphs.

Harnessing Hyper-Focus

Another superpower of ADHD—hyper-focus—plays a significant role in turning challenges into achievements. Many women with ADHD report experiencing bursts of intense focus, where they can become completely immersed in a task. While this can lead to difficulties in shifting attention, it can also result in unparalleled productivity in areas that ignite passion.

Sophie often advised her clients on how to channel hyper-focus effectively. "Identify what excites you and lean into it," she suggested. "Set aside time where you can fully engage with the work you love without distractions." Over time, she developed a system where she allowed specific times for hyper-focusing on her artistic projects while establishing breaks to prevent burnout.

In the creative arts, this focused energy can yield truly remarkable results. Artists report producing some of their best work during these periods, creating art that reflects not only their experiences but also their unique perspectives. Hyper-focus, when understood and embraced, can enhance both the creative process and the final product.

Concluding Thoughts: Your ADHD Narrative

As the chapter draws to a close, Sophie encourages readers to rewrite their ADHD narratives. Instead of viewing their diagnosis as a limitation, they can begin to see it as a unique aspect of their identities—one that comes with distinctive strengths. The journey to embrace one's superpowers is not without struggle, and women may face societal pressures that undermine their self-worth, but the process of self-acceptance creates an empowering pathway to personal and professional success.

"Every woman with ADHD has the potential to be extraordinary," Sophie affirms. "It's about finding your strengths and using them to carve out a unique place in the world."

In her vibrant studio, surrounded by the creative chaos she has cultivated, Sophie embodies this belief. She is a testament to the idea that ADHD, rather than a barrier, can indeed be a superpower—an integral part of an inspiring journey defined by resilience, creativity, and an unwavering determination to thrive. Let this chapter encourage readers to discover and celebrate their own superpowers, forging a brighter future defined by their newfound strengths.

www.ingramcontent.com/pod-product-compliance
Lightning Source LLC
Chambersburg PA
CBHW071727020426
42333CB00017B/2430